LOVE YOURSELF AND INTERMITTENT FASTING

21 Day Plan for Learning "Self-Love" and 7 effective techniques of Intermittent Fasting

Stephen Fleming

Love Yourself and Intermittent Fasting

Copyright © 2017 Stephen Fleming

All rights reserved.

Love Yourself and Intermittent Fasting

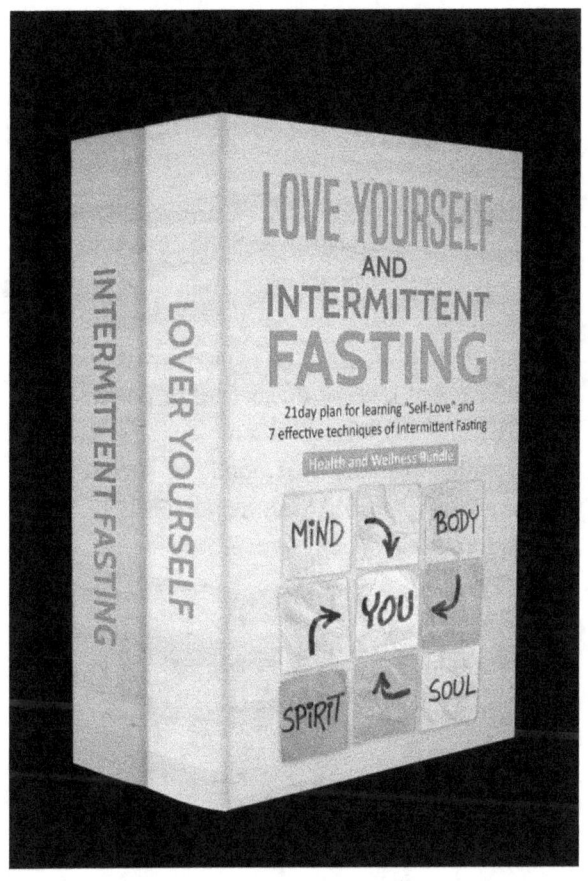

Welcome On-Board: Get the FREE BONUS

I am privileged to have you onboard. You have shown faith in me and I would like to reciprocate it by offering the maximum value with an amazing gift.

As you are working towards improving your life consistently, I would like to contribute in your journey by offering a free bonus called "Health & Wealth Magnetism- Using the law of attraction to create Health & Wealth". It provides an interesting perspective to overall success and how health & wealth compliments each other to create a lasting success. I would be adding to this free bonus as I find other beneficial topics that can help contribute in our progress.

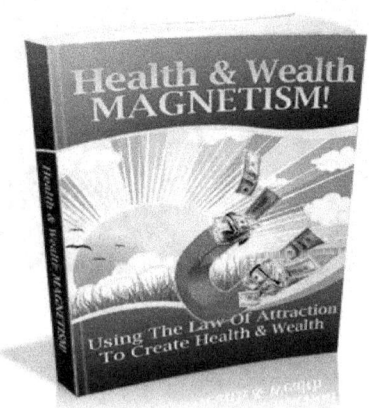

Love Yourself and Intermittent Fasting

Type this link: http://eepurl.com/dglqCH
or scan below from your mobile

Love Yourself and Intermittent Fasting

© Copyright 2017 - All rights reserved.

This document is geared towards providing exact and reliable information in regards to the topic and issue covered. The publication is sold with the idea that the publisher is not required to render accounting, officially permitted, or otherwise, qualified services. If advice is necessary, legal or professional, a practiced individual in the profession should be ordered.

- From a Declaration of Principles which was accepted and approved equally by a Committee of the American Bar Association and a Committee of Publishers and Associations.

In no way is it legal to reproduce, duplicate, or transmit any part of this document in either electronic means or in printed format. Recording of this publication is strictly prohibited and any storage of this document is not allowed unless with written permission from the publisher. All rights reserved.

The information provided herein is stated to be truthful and consistent, in that any liability, in terms of inattention or otherwise, by any usage or abuse of any policies, processes, or directions contained within is the solitary and utter responsibility of the recipient reader. Under no circumstances will any legal responsibility or blame be held against the publisher for any reparation, damages, or monetary loss due to the information herein, either directly or indirectly.

Respective authors own all copyrights not held by the publisher.

The information herein is offered for informational purposes solely, and is universal as so. The presentation of the information is without contract or any type of guarantee assurance.

The trademarks that are used are without any consent, and the publication of the trademark is without permission or backing by the trademark owner. All trademarks and brands within this book are for clarifying purposes only and are the owned by the owners themselves, not affiliated with this document.

BOOK 1:

LOVE YOURSELF:

21 Day Plan for Learning "Self-Love" To Cultivate Self-Worth, Self-Belief, Self-Confidence, Happiness

1	Introduction	1
2	Understanding Self Love	2-6
3	21 Day action plan for learning the art of Self Love	7-36

1. INTRODUCTION

I want to thank you and congratulate you for downloading the book, "Love yourself - 21 Day Plan for Learning "Self-Love" To Cultivate Self-Worth, Self-Belief, Self-Confidence, Happiness".

Self-love greatly affects how we see ourselves. It affects how much we value ourselves. When you practice self-love, you see yourself as valuable and understand your worth; this helps you know you deserve respect and appreciation. As unfortunate as it sounds, we live in a world where society has led us into believing that the best measure for self-worth is in terms of wealth, status, careers, sex, and power. In the real sense however, measuring yourself against these traits only raises more feelings of being inadequate. You end up immersing yourself in unending self-loathing. Learning to practice self-love will help you conquer this feeling and negativity. To understand why you need self-love, you need to know what self-love is first. This guide will teach you everything you need to know about self-love. In this book, you will learn the difference between narcissism and self-love and how to love yourself unconditionally so that you can live a happier and fulfilling life. Thanks for downloading and enjoy the ride.

2. UNDERSTANDING SELF-LOVE

Self-love is an unconditional feeling of love and appreciation towards you. In our day-to-day life, we often have to deal with situations that cause us to look at ourselves from a 'we are failures perspective'. This especially happens when we fail to attain a specific goal. Self-love in this case is greatly valuing you despite your weaknesses, failures, and shortcomings. Self-love does not mean that you are oblivious of your mistakes or weaknesses but rather you know that as a human being you will fail and being bold enough to love and appreciate yourself despite this.

Before we start learning how to practice self-love, let us understand how you stand to benefit by practicing self-love.

How You Benefit From Loving Yourself Unconditionally

Practicing self-love has the following benefits:

Helps you accept any outcome: When you

practice self-love, you know you are worth and deserve respect; thus, you learn to accept yourself through everything.

When you fully love and accept yourself, you recognize rejection or negative outcome from a given activity as a redirection to take a different route. Instead of beating yourself up over a failure or rejection, you accept the situation, learn from it, and move on with your life. Negative outcomes do not devastatingly affect you because you greatly value yourself and you do not attach the value on any particular outcome.

You learn how to accept yourself: When you love who you are, you accept whom you are. After learning how to practice self-love, you become aware of your strengths and weaknesses, and learn to accept both of them by realizing how unique you are. You stop seeking to be what you are not and instead learn to accept who you are and then start working on becoming the person you want to be.

Helps you deal with negativity from others: As you practice self-love, the opinions of those around you (especially when that opinion is negative) stops bearing immense value. The value you place on their opinions reasonably decreases.

You evaluate the things you spend your time on and discover things that are most important to you. With this, you gain confidence that what you are doing matters, which helps you hold less value to what people consider to matter to you.

Increases your self-confidence: Practicing self-love helps improve our inner voice and power. When you practice self-love, you tune your inner voice to positivity. This helps boost your confidence. You also focus on your positive traits, which boosts your self-confidence and charisma.

Enables you to set clear priorities: After practicing self-love, you become conscious of how you spend your time and the things you spend it on. With this awareness, your priorities change and you align yourself with what you deem most important. You evaluate everything you are spending your time on and when you realize you are spending your time on things that don't matter much, you change accordingly.

Increases the amount of love we receive

from others: This is because after practicing self-love, you recognize what love is. You learn to focus on the positive aspects of every person and cut people some slack knowing that just like you, they have weaknesses. This increases the feeling of mutual love. It also helps increase your ability to accept love offered by others by accepting you are lovable **and making** you able to recognize love and accept love offered to you.

Makes us happier: After practicing self-love, you accept that you have flaws. With this understanding, you can work on improving your flaws as well as your strengths. For the things you cannot change, you accept that you are not perfect and this realization enables you not to hold on what you cannot do. This is likely to make you a happier person.

You understand yourself better: Self-love helps you understand yourself. It also helps you learn the things that matter to you and enables you to understand why you make mistakes and how each aspect of your life triggers different emotions within you.

By practicing self-love, you learn to appreciate your flaws and work on your strengths to make yourself a better person.

As you have read above, by practicing self-love, you stand to benefit greatly. However, in order to start enjoying these benefits, you first need to learn how to practice self-love. Learning how to practice self-love is a process and to practice self-love, you have to go through various steps. Following is a 21-day guide to practicing self-love.

3. 21 DAY ACTION PLAN FOR LEARNING THE ART OF SELF LOVE

The following are day-to-day steps you have to follow to learn how to practice self-love. At the end of this 21-day self-love action plan, you should be in a position where you can effortlessly practice self-love and derive all the benefits it brings with it:

Day 1-7: Laying the Foundation

In the next seven days, you will be laying the foundation you need to practice immense self-love.

Day 1: Understanding Self-Love

The first step to learning how to love you is having an understanding of what self-love is. Understanding what self-love is will help you know why you need it. Therefore, the first step is defining self-love from a personal perspective.

How to do it

1. The first thing you need to do is determine

if you have been practicing self-love. You can do this by listing the normal life situations you go through that can show if you appreciate yourself and if you find yourself worthy. For example, consider the following questions:

Do the negative things people say to you get to you?

Do you beat yourself too hard when you fail to achieve your goals?

Do you do things that matter to you?

Can you tune out negative energy from the outside world?

If you realize you have not been practicing self-love, find a strong 'why' for why you should practice self-love. How will self-love help you? Revisit the benefits of self-love and make a short list of those that ring true to you. This will motivate you to learn how to practice self-love.

2. The second thing you need to do is understand the dangers of not practicing self-love. Learning the dangers of lacking self-love will remind you 'why' self-love is important. Lack of self-love can lead to harmful choices that include the following:

*It can lead to reliance on other people's opinions for validation.

*It can also lead to deprivation of happiness. When you lack self-love, you tend to absorb all the negative energy around you. This ends up blocking your happiness

*Lack of self-love also hinders emotional healing. To be happy, you have to forgive yourself for any wrong doings. A lack of self-love prevents this.

3. The third thing you have to do is understand the existence of negative energy in the outside world. This will help you understand the necessity of self-love. Understand that although you may hear negative comments from other people, this should not set you off.

Realize the need to learn to brush off this negative energy without letting it bruise your feelings. Identify the need to learn how to practice self-love and recognize your readiness to learn how to do it. Prepare yourself psychologically for this process and be ready to learn.

Day 2: Getting To Know Yourself
Getting to know yourself will help you know

your strengths. In return, this will help you see why you are worthy and deserving of appreciation. It will boost how you see yourself and the value you attach to yourself.

How to do it

Dedicate five minutes to focusing on yourself: Give yourself the gift of time. Do not feel as if you are wasting this time; enjoy the moment. Take a journal and list your strengths and positive attributes. This process may be hard if for a long time, you have been continuously looking down upon yourself. Just take your time to find something positive in your life. This could include the following:

I am a friendly and sociable person.

I am a good time manager

I can think on my feet

I am innovative

I have a big heart that seeks to help those in difficulties

I am bright and smart

While making this list, ensure you are specific.

Do not use general adjectives. For instance, instead of writing "I am caring" you can write the following "Each time I see someone struggling, I take time to know what that person is going through and do my level best to help that person out."

When you finish creating the list, go through your points. However minor they may be, understand that each single one of them is a clear reason why you deserve love and respect.

After listing your points, rise up and go to the mirror. Take your time to look at the image staring back at you. Absorb what you are seeing. Admire the person staring back at you, look yourself in the eyes, and tell yourself that 'you love you.' Self-admiration will boost your confidence.

Go to work and if during the day, anything happens that might pull you back to self-loathing, recite the "I love you" mantra. This will help clear your negative thoughts. At the end of the day, take time to reevaluate

yourself. Take note of how you feel. Set a goal to write each positive aspect in your life. This will help you know your progress.

Day 3: Improving Your Inner Voice

Improving your inner voice will help you tune off negativity by creating positive affirmations against the negative thoughts you may have.

How to do it

1. Stand up and assume a comfortable posture. Focus on your general feeling and how you are feeling; are you relaxed or do you feel energetic? Tune your concentration to breathing and focus on the sequence of your breaths. This will help you become attentive.

2. Understand today's focus as 'improving your inner voice.' Try to understand what your inner voice does to you. This will help you understand why you need to work on improving your inner voice.

Our inner voice affects how we see ourselves and how we see others. Identify the need to improve your inner voice, write down the ways you can do it, and expound on each one of them. This may include the following:

Overcoming negative beliefs about yourself

*Avoiding perfectionism

*Discarding your negative filter

Love Yourself and Intermittent Fasting

*Focusing on the positive aspects of your life

Understand the existence of negative energy both from within yourself and from the outside world. This will help you understand why you need to improve your inner voice.

Determine if you hold any negative beliefs about yourself. You can do this by asking yourself these questions.

Do you ever have regrets about something in your past?

Do you hate yourself for lacking a certain thing or trait?

Do you ever feel like you are not good enough? You may hate yourself for a mistake or failure you made in the past.

Identify how these beliefs and thoughts affect you in your daily life. This will help you understand why you need to shower yourself with self-love.

3. Find out if you work towards perfection. This will help you see how perfectionism

affects your general life. Find out how you feel when you are less than perfect. Understand the effort you put in your daily life activities even if you fail to attain your expected perfection. This will help you learn self-appreciation even on minor things. Promise yourself to consider the effort you put into something rather than focusing on the outcome.

4. Discard your negative filter by focusing only on the positive things in your life rather than the negative ones. Try to look at everything in your life from a different perspective: a better perspective. This improves your psychological and emotional state by creating positivity in everything. Even when everything seems to be going wrong, try to find a single positive aspect you can focus on.

5. Rewrite your internal script. When you notice you have negative thoughts about yourself, accept these thoughts first, and then try to determine their source, before moving on to rewriting each negative thought with a positive one. For example, if you forget to buy something you needed, accept that you forgot to buy sugar, but understand you are a human being prone to mistakes. This will tune your mind into having a positive approach on each matter, which will help get rid of general negativity in your life.

6. At the end of the day, take time to reevaluate yourself. This will help you notice if you are making any progress. Take note of how you feel. Did you notice any other positive aspect in your life? Add it to the previous list – this will grow your list of why you are worthy and deserving of appreciation.

Day 4: Recognizing Love

What does love feel like? Recognizing love will help you know whether you have been practicing self-love and know when you are practicing self-love.

How to do it

Start your day with mindful breathing. Close your eyes and focus your thoughts on the sequence of your breaths. Take a slow deep breath then exhale slowly. This will help heighten your concentration. Take note of your today's point of focus

As stated earlier, understanding what love is or being able to recognize these feelings may be quite difficult if you have been constantly looking down on yourself.

Practicing loving-kindness mindfulness will help you unveil the feelings of love. It will equip you with tools you need to practice self-love. Below is how to practice loving-kindness mindfulness.

1. Assume a comfortable sitting posture.

2. Focus your concentration on your breathing, take a slow deep breath, and then slowly exhale it. This will help you focus on your breathing.

3. As you continue breathing, create positive affirmations that you will repeat in your mind. Identify any negative feelings or thoughts you may incur after reciting each affirmation and identify their **source.**

4. Think of yourself. Identify the feelings that come along with thinking about you. If any negative thoughts arise, replace them with positive affirmations.

Day 5: Becoming Emotionally Honest

We often fake how we feel in order to be accepted. Emotional dishonesty is one of the threats to practicing self-love and achieving happiness. It is also one of the reasons why you think you are not good enough. You cannot be happy if you are not honest with your emotions. Emotional honesty helps you break the circle of fear and build one of self-appreciation by enabling you to know your true self.

How to do it

1. Start your day with mindful breathing. Close your eyes, take a deep slow breath, and then slowly exhale it. Take note of the changes occurring on and within your body as you breathe. This will help you focus on the current situation. Take note of today's point of focus.

2. Identify times in your life when you have been emotionally dishonest with yourself; such as the time you lied to yourself about how you feel about liking a person you dislike or feeling sad but acting happy. This will help you realize the negative effects of emotional dishonesty.

3. Identify why you try to numb your feelings and what you do to numb them. Perhaps you try to numb your feelings so you can act strong or feel strong and you may be numbing your feelings by getting drunk, binge shopping, or engaging in other unhealthy behaviors.

4. Try to understand the need for emotional honesty by revisiting its benefits that include fostering courage, creating connection, and eliminating garbage. This will give you the motivation to be honest with yourself. Set an intention to be emotionally honest with

yourself today henceforth.

5. During the day, identify various emotions you experience during that day; this could be hatred or sadness. Find out if you have been emotionally honest with yourself. For the negative emotions, find their source, and then try developing a way to curb them.

For example, you can find out why you hate a person or thing, and then start seeking ways to stop hating it or them. You may choose to focus on a single positive aspect in the beginning. This will help unveil other positive aspects.

At the end of the day, take time to reevaluate yourself to see if you have adhered to the previous steps. This will help you note your progress.

Day 6: Becoming Real

Being real is one of the things we struggle with in our day-to-day lives. Sometimes we hide our true selves to avoid being hurt again. Even so, being real helps build trust in ourselves. To become real, we need to understand its benefits. This will act as the motivation that will encourage you to practice self-love. The benefits of being real include:

Compassion: Being real helps us learn how to be compassionate towards ourselves. Speaking our minds helps us love ourselves and able to achieve the outcome we desire.

Bravery: Being true to yourself teaches you to be courageous and strong. When you are true to yourself, you let others know when you do not approve of something without fear of judgment or rejection.

Comfort: When you openly express yourself, you become comfortable knowing some weight is now off your chest.

Positivity: Learning to trust your inner voice helps you realize the benefit of being real. This motivates you to surround yourself with people who encourage you to be your true self, which ends up building positivity.

How to be real

1. Start by mindful breathing. Take a slow deep breath then exhale slowly. This will help bring your focus to what you are doing. Take note of the topic you will base your focus on today.

2. Identify the number of times you have been

real and spoken out your mind and feelings. Identify how this made you feel. Did it boost your confidence? How did it make you feel? This will help you understand the need to be real. Once you do this, implement the following steps:

*Maintain a journal where you write your feelings; write down the various experiences you experience in life and whether you spoke your mind in each of them. This will act as an encouragement to speak up your mind whenever the chance presents itself.

*Practice mirror work; learn to create a similar image of the feelings inside you by speaking out exactly how you feel

*Set the intention for that day as speaking your mind. If you do not approve of something, make it known. This will boost your confidence and help boost your happiness.

*At the end of the day, reevaluate yourself to see if you have adhered to your previous steps. This will help you know if you are making any progress.

Day 7: Protect Yourself

Protecting yourself means eliminating all the negative energy surrounding you. If you keep the company of people who keep looking down on you or degrading you, it slows your healing process and progress towards practicing self-love. For this reason, you need to do something about all the negative people and stimuli around you.

How to learn to protect yourself

1. Start each process by mindful breathing. Take a slow deep breath and then exhale slowly. Do this for five minutes and take note of the changes occurring in your body as you do this. This will help heighten your concentration on what you are doing. Take note of your today's point of focus.

2. Identify people in your life who create negative energy. For instance, consider people who say negative things that really hurt you. Identify the emotions these people cause. This will help you realize the need to protect yourself from such characters.

3. Understand the need to get rid of them. There is not enough time in your life to spend time on people who drain you of your happiness. Therefore, detach from anyone you feel is a threat to your happiness.

Day 8-14: Continuity

Here is what you shall be doing for the next 7 days:

Day 8: Identify Your Priorities

Identifying the things that matter to you will help you know what you need to focus on to increase your happiness.

How to identify your priorities

1. Start your day with mindful breathing. Take a slow deep breath then slowly exhale. Take note of the changes occurring in your body, as you do this. For example, notice the rise and fall of your chest. Once you are mindful, identify your point of focus for the day.

2. Create a list of things that matter to you. Ask yourself this question; what do I value most? Create a list of all things that matter most to you.

3. Understand the need to avoid participating in negativity-laced activities that pull you down. This will help boost your self-confidence. Participating in activities that tamper with your happiness promotes feelings of inadequacy. You should therefore work towards avoiding such activities. Instead, from

today onwards, only do things that you enjoy.

At the end of the day, evaluate yourself and determine if you adhered to your principles, and if you did not, do not scold yourself. Accept it and commit to being better next time. Reevaluating yourself will help you see if you are making progress.

Day 9: Forgive Yourself

Forgiveness is a major step towards learning self-appreciation and self-love. We often scold ourselves and hate ourselves for our past failures and mistakes. We cannot love ourselves if we keep looking down on ourselves. To practice self-love, you thereby need to take a step towards forgiving yourself.

How to forgive yourself

1. Start with mindful breathing. Take a deep slow breath then slowly let it out. Take note of the changes occurring in your body as you do this. This will help heighten your concentration. Once you are calm, you can focus on today's task.

2. Accept you have made several mistakes in your life. This will help you reconcile with yourself. Denying that you have failed will only

make the healing process more difficult. 3. Create a list of the various mistakes you have made so far in your life. This could include the following:

*Failing your exams

*Not qualifying for a promotion at work

4. Understand that you are a human being and that you are prone to making mistakes. Learn to take failures as opportunities to learn. If you fail to achieve something, take it as a chance to learn to be better in your next encounter. This will help reduce the hatred you feel towards yourself for your failures.

To better your life, allow yourself to look past your mistakes. You can do this by looking into each of your past failure and concentrating on the effort you exerted as you tried to achieve something better.

For example, for failing in your exams, take note of the effort you put into studying. Appreciate yourself for that. From this day henceforth, set the intention of focusing on your current life and look past your failures.

Day 10: Become Mindful

Mindfulness is a state of awareness whereby

you take note of emotions, feelings, and everything around you. Mindfulness is one of the key steps towards practicing self-love and self-appreciation. When you are mindful, you become aware of what you want, feel, or think.

This helps you in a number of ways that include like enabling you take note of degrading thoughts and redirecting them. You also become mindful of who you are and able to use this knowledge to be what you **want to be** rather than what others want for you.

How to become mindful

1. Take a slow deep breath then slowly let it out. Take note of the changes occurring in your body as you do this.

2. Identify the need of mindfulness in your life. Ask yourself this question; how does mindfulness benefit me? Revisit the benefits of mindfulness. This will act as motivation to practice mindfulness.

3. Try identifying the times in your life when you practiced mindfulness. How did this help you? This will help you know why you need to practice mindfulness. Set that day and each day after to be mindful of everything you are doing.

4. At the end of the day, reevaluate yourself to see if you have adhered to what you had set to. This will help you know if you are progressing towards your end goal: self-love.

Day 11: Discover The Power Of Fun

Having fun will enable you to loosen up. Engage in activities that are fun and ones that boost your mood. When you are happy, you are very unlikely to fall back to looking down on yourself and focusing on your failures or weaknesses. You instead focus on the brighter side of life, which boosts your happiness.

How to have fun

1. Understand the benefits fun brings with it: list the benefits of having fun. This may include the following:

Having fun boosts confidence: confidence is very central to building self-love. Fun helps boost the level of endorphins in the body. Endorphins act as neurotransmitters that send message of confidence and satisfaction to the brain. This in return results in a more cheerful and self-assured you.

Having fun is also good for de-stressing. When you are having fun, you focus on the positive side of life rather than the negative one. A hobby helps you experience what life has to offer.

2. Identify fun activities you can engage in; this could be swimming or dancing. Once you have this, set out to engage in these activities and while at them, enjoy yourself. This will increase your happiness and positively change how you see yourself.

3. At the end of the day, evaluate yourself and assess how you feel. Determine if you have adhered to the previous steps. You can create a list of all the steps then tick besides each item if you have adhered to them and place a cross next to the ones you have not adhered to. This will help you take note of your progress.

Day 12: Live In Appreciation

Appreciation is being grateful for everything in your life. It involves celebrating your victories no matter how small or big they are, embracing things that make you different by understanding that they are what makes you special, appreciating every single positive aspect in your life ranging from beauty, talents, and brilliance. Practicing appreciation enables you to love your imperfectly perfect self. It reminds you why you are worth.

How to be grateful

1. Try to understand the benefits of

appreciation. This will act as motivation for you to practice appreciation. The benefits of appreciation include:

It boosts your self-esteem - It makes you able to focus on the positive aspects, which boosts your self-esteem.

Enables you achieve goals faster; appreciation increases determination, energy, and enthusiasm, which all act as driving tools towards achieving your goals.

2. Make a list of your strengths and victories and then take time to look into each one of them. This will remind you why you are worthy. For each day, look at this list; it will motivate you to live each day to the **fullest. It is inevitable not to have down days; therefore, learn to find something** positive about each day and focus on this positive.

Day 13: Setting Limits

We live in a busy world where our commitments are immeasurable. Because of this, we often lose track of our limits. It is thereby necessary to set limits about how much we can do in a particular day without wearing ourselves out. This will help you take better care of yourself.

How to set limits

1. Identify things that matter to you. Setting a clear list of your priorities will help you know what you need to do and what you need to say no to. You will love yourself more when you say no to activities or work that deprives you of your happiness, emotional and physical wellbeing.

2. You can do this by doing the following:

Set a strict schedule for waking up and going to sleep.

Make a list of your commitments for the day.

Set a limit on how many hours you need to work in a day.

Day 14: Practice Good Self-Care

When you nourish your body well, you love and appreciate yourself more. Let us look at how to practice good self-care:

How to practice good self-care

*Look at yourself in the mirror and admire your image. You can tell yourself how pretty you look that day or any other positive thing that pops into your mind. This will act as a reminder of why you need to take good care of your body and self.

*Learn to eat a healthy balanced diet. It is also advisable to exercise.

*Practice good hygiene and groom yourself appropriately

As you take care of your mind to get rid of negative thoughts and beliefs, you also need to take good care of your body. The more you practice good self-care, the more you boost your confidence, the more you feel good about yourself and the more you will love yourself.

Day 15-21: Last Leg

Here is what you shall be doing in the last seven days of the 21-day self-love action plan:

Day 15: Avoid Comparisons

Comparing yourself to people is one of the sources of self-loathing. When you do not possess traits other people seem to have, you tend to think that others are better than you while in real sense, being different from the rest of the crowd is what makes us special. Therefore, there is a need to get rid of these comparisons.

How to do this

Create a list of traits you possess that the people around you do not have. This can include the following:

*Generosity

*Patience

*Understanding

Include even the minor traits you have. Look into the benefits of having each of these traits. Concentrating on these traits will remind you of how special you are for being different.

Day 16: Learning Patience
Learning self-love is a process. Self-love is something we need to practice daily but as unfortunate as it sounds, self-love can take long to master, which is why you need to practice patience. Practicing patience boosts self-acceptance and appreciation.

How to practice patience

You can do this by understanding that self-love is a process. This will help you improve the patience you have towards yourself. Therefore, mastering this will take more than a day.

To make the process easier, eliminate the fear

and urgency to learn to do it. You can do this by:

Understanding that change is a hard and long process: you cannot change overnight. Accepting this will help you understand why you need to be patient with yourself.

Understanding the importance of pressing on. Remind yourself why you need this by revisiting the <u>benefits of self-love</u>.

Day 17: Live Intentionally

You will love yourself more when you have a strong purpose. When you set a goal you need to achieve, upon achieving it, you appreciate yourself more and love yourself deeper.

How to live intentionally

Set a goal or purpose you need to achieve. This could be living a meaningful and healthy life and then work towards achieving this goal. For example, ensure you eat nutritious meals so you can maintain your health. After a while, evaluate whether you have attained your goal or objective. If you have, you will feel better and love yourself more for attaining such simple goals.

Day 18: Follow Your Passion

Your passion is what you love doing and you would not mind doing it if someone work you up in the middle of the night. Following your passion will boost your self-esteem and boost your moods.

How to follow your passion

Identify things that excite you; this could be drawing or writing, and then set an intention to involve yourself in any of your given activities. Do the things you like but are scared to engage in. In the end, doing these things will boost your confidence and self-esteem, which are key ingredients to practicing self-love.

Day 19: Accept Uncertainty

We live in fear of what the future may hold and constantly allow pain from our past to predict our future and torment our present life. To learn self-love, you need to understand and accept that uncertainty is part of everyday life.

How to accept uncertainty

Let go of your past traumas. To do this, create a list of previous experiences that rob you of your inner peace and torment you. Look into each of them, accept that they happened, and you can do nothing to change them.

Instead of letting them torment you, use them as a learning platform for your betterment. Understand that there exists uncertainty on what the future may hold, but always hope for the best and live in the moment. This will help you attain a state of peace.

Day 20: Let Go Of What You Cannot Change

Some situations in our lives are beyond our ability to alter. To be at peace with yourself, learn to let go of such things otherwise, they will deprive you of the joy of living in the moment.

How to Do this

To let go, you need to look at different situations in your life. Accept the way everything in your life is. For instance, accept your current economic situation; this, however, should not be an excuse to be lazy but rather to be realistic with the situation and the options available to you to make the necessary changes Stop fighting with yourself or wishing things were different; accept where you are and work with what you have to become better.

Day 21: Follow Your Inner Voice

To practice self-love, you need to follow your conscience. When you follow your conscience in undertaking various activities in your life, you gain satisfaction from the results.

How to do this

When you are confused about which choices to make or the path to follow in your life, take a moment, take a deep breath and listen to your conscience. There is always that inner voice guiding us on what to do. Follow it when making choices. Following your deeper small inner voice boosts your confidence and self-esteem. It also helps us accept all the outcomes whatsoever.

Conclusion

Thank you again for purchasing this book!

As you implement this 21-day self-love action plan, also try something new as often as you can out of your normal schedule. For example, if you create specified meals each day of the week, choose to step out of your comfort zone and try a new recipe or add some more spices. See how this works for you. You will feel more satisfied with yourself for making this new discovery: self-satisfaction leads to self-love.

....

Hey! Do you mind giving your feedback on Amazon by rating and reviewing my book.

I would really appreciate that.

....

BOOK 2:

INTERMITTENT FASTING:
7 Effective Techniques with Scientific Approach To Stay Healthy, Lose Weight, Slow Down Aging Process & Live Longer

1	Introduction	38-39
2	Intermittent Fasting Explained	40-43
3	Scientific Logic Behind Intermittent Fasting	44-46
4	Benefits of Intermittent Fasting	47-50
5	Intermittent Fasting Techniques	51-64
6	Tips to Succeed with Fasting & Conclusion	65-68

1. INTRODUCTION

I want to thank you and congratulate you for downloading the book, "Intermittent Fasting - 7 Effective Techniques with Scientific Approach To Stay Healthy, Lose Weight, Slow Down Aging Process & Live Longer"

Did you know that human beings have been fasting since evolution? Basically, human beings mainly fasted due to lack of food and for a number of reasons. For instance, both the ancient man and the hunter-gatherers didn't have food stores or refrigerators to make food available all-year round. In some instances, these people never found anything to eat and their body nevertheless "evolved" to function without food for long periods!

On the other hand, there are religions among them Christians, Islam, and Buddhists who embrace fasting as part of the doctrine. This clearly shows that fasting is not something new. However, how can you exactly fast to lose weight? This is what this book will be about.

This book will teach you about intermittent fasting, how to lose weight with intermittent fasting, why intermittent fasting is effective at weight loss, 7 techniques of intermittent fasting and so much more.

Thanks again for downloading this book. I hope you enjoy it!

2. INTERMITTENT FASTING EXPLAINED

Intermittent fasting refers to a pattern of eating that alternates between periods of fasting and non-fasting, intended to facilitate weight loss or boost health. For starters, intermittent fasting does not restrict foods or calories to eat but rather suggests when you should eat them.

There are different approaches to intermittent fasting with some involving calorie restriction, skipping some meals and total fasting. For instance, during the fasting period, you can eat limited amounts of low-calories foods or drinks such as tea or coffee. Alternatively, you may choose to reduce intake of calories say to 20 percent on fasting days rather than not eating altogether. If desired, you can also choose to fast for a complete 24 hours then eat normally for the next 24 hours in what is called alternate day fasting.

Due to these flexibilities, it's easier to adopt a favorite dieting plan by deciding the number of hours or days to fast and activities to carry out during the fast. But with too much freedom, how does intermittent fasting work? Basically, you should understand what happens to your body during the eating phase and the fasted state.

Once you eat, your body is said to be at a fed state where it's digesting and assimilating food and nutrients. The fed state normally commences once you start to eat, and often lasts for 3-5 hours. In this state, it's harder to burn fat due to high levels of insulin.

Insulin is a hormone that facilitates uptake of glucose into body cells. After a high carb meal, glucose level increases which triggers high concentration of insulin. As the hormone only helps glucose uptake, your body has to utilize glucose for energy rather than stored fats.

After the action of insulin, the body goes into post-absorption state where no food is processed, a period that lasts for 8-12 hours after a meal. Then you enter into a fasted state about 12 hours after your last meal, where insulin level is significantly reduced. In a fasted state, it's easier to burn fat that was inaccessible during the period of eating. While there are different intermittent fasting techniques, there are common guidelines applicable across board. Let us look at these guidelines in the following chapter.

Intermittent Fasting Guidelines

According to research, even eating three meals a day can be "eating too much" as far as calorie restriction and meal planning is concerned. The study found out that eating fewer meals a day could be better than increased meal frequency particularly in the long term.

While eating 5-6 smaller meals a day can help control blood sugar and curb hunger, your metabolism often is accustomed to the schedule within 1-2 months. Later on you start experiencing hunger throughout the day rather than around lunch or dinnertime.

A better approach is to embrace intermittent fasting and limit meals to a narrow window of 8 hours ideally by skipping breakfast. To make it easier, choose to either eat breakfast or dinner but not both. For instance you could choose to eat a solid breakfast and lunch if working in a physically taxing job and then skip dinner. The great thing is that it actually doesn't matter what meal you skip as long as you skip one of the meals.

The rule of the thumb is to only eat within a window of 6-8 consecutive hours daily and then eat meals at least 3 hours before bed. While you can still fast for 24 hours, skipping just a few meals can optimize your mitochondrial function and inhibit any cellular

damage. You don't have to starve yourself but rather eat enough food while allowing the body to rest from constant feeding

In the following chapter, we are going to look at the scientific logic behind intermittent fasting and its effectiveness.

3. SCIENTIFIC LOGIC BEHIND INTERMITTENT FASTING

Whether you simply take coffee for breakfast in place of high-fructose fruit smoothie or skip breakfast altogether, you gain in terms of improved health and weight loss. And while lack of food may be thought to trigger breakdown of muscle, your body first breaks down stored glycogen into glucose to fuel metabolic activities. Once glycogen levels are depleted, the body begins to break down stored fat for energy. In some cases, excess amino acids from proteins can be metabolized for energy though this does not mean the body may break down muscle.

Most people against intermittent fasting state that it reduces your metabolism because your body thinks that you are starving; hence, slowing down, which can make weight loss impossible. However, this is not the case. According to research, the rate of metabolism doesn't change when you enter into a fasting state as long as you don't exceed 60 hours. However, even after 60 hours of continuous fasting, the study found out that the rate of metabolism only reduced by a mere 8 percent. Actually, to some extent, the rate of metabolism can significantly be speeded up after 36-48 hours of fasting according to related research. This is because when you fast, the brain releases chemicals or neurotransmitters such as adrenaline and noradrenalin. These help activate your mind and basal metabolic rate (BMR) which serves to facilitate you to work or go to search for food. This can continue until 72 hours of total fasting, where the body opts to break down muscle as primary source of energy. In addition to a boosted metabolism, other studies reveal that the intermittent fasting helps boost energy production, memory, and cognitive function. Furthermore, it can boost production of proteins that stimulates neuron growth and protection. This is referred to as neurotrophic growth factor.

Another study found out that intermittent fasting could reduce insulin resistance. An increase in insulin sensitivity and reduced blood pressure help control diseases such as stroke and coronary artery disease. Intermittent fasting can also boost resistance of the heart and brain cells to ischemic injury that causes diseases such as stroke. In a related research, believers who undertake Ramadan fasting were found to have reduced risk to diabetes, improved immunity and cardiovascular health. Though this study was based on short-term achievements, it's agreed that intermittent fasting is a great thing to try out.

If intending to lose weight or burn fat, a certain study found out that fasting boosts the activity in genes that burn calories and stored body fat. When fasting, the body activates genes that encode enzymes and uncoupling proteins that increase fat oxidation. These proteins "poke holes" into mitochondria (body cells that make energy) and this reduces the overall amount of energy generated. As a result, the body has to burn more fat or calories to achieve the same amount of energy.

Better still; further studies suggest that intermittent fasting can help your cells to handle stress. When you stop eating, body cells are jolted into a minor stressful state, which strengthens them to fight other stresses that often lead to disease.

From the scientific studies, it's obvious that intermittent fasting can help you lose weight, boost cardiovascular health and help you live longer. Let's learn more about these benefits and other benefits of intermittent fasting.

4. BENEFITS OF INTERMITTENT FASTING

Intermittent fasting boasts of benefits such as weight loss, slowing down aging and prolonging your life. Whatever your intended reason for intermittent fasting, you can enjoy a number of benefits like:

1: Weight loss

As already pointed out above, research has shown that people who eat a single meal daily rather than the usual 3 meals lose more weight and have more muscle. This is because dieters who adopt intermittent fasting eat less frequently, actually feel hungry less, and are more likely to feel fuller after eating.

Intermittent fasting can also help you enter a fat burning state referred to as ketosis. When fasting, you deplete your body of glucose, its main source of energy, and this forces the body to break down stored fats for energy. Furthermore, adding MCT oil in coffee during fasting days helps speed up the ketosis process, and yields higher ketones, which fuel the brain.

That's not all; intermittent fasting can be used

as a calorie restriction strategy where you fast for 24 hours at least twice per week. If you follow this eating pattern, you reduce your calorie intake by around 30 percent and thus make it easier to lose weight. By taking in lesser

calories, you force the body to utilize stored glycogen and body fats for energy, a situation that facilitates weight loss.

2: Better hormonal function

Intermittent fasting helps improve your body composition and boosts functionality of hormones. More importantly, you become more sensitive to insulin hormone especially if you pair fasting with exercise. A controlled insulin level helps reduce blood sugar, suppress hunger, and fight occasional food cravings. In addition, research shows that by fasting intermittently for around 40 hours, you also boost the production of growth hormone (GH) up to 5-folds. This hormone has many benefits among them speeding up the rate of fat loss and muscle gain. The growth hormone also helps offset the effects of cortisol, a stress hormone that affects fat storage at the belly.

3: Living longer

Research shows that intermittent fasting can prolong your lifespan in a similar manner as a calorie-restricted diet. This study has found out that reducing your calorie consumption by about 30-40 percent can help extend life at least by 33 percent. Further research shows that fasting can offer health benefits against diabetes, cancer, cardiovascular problems, and Alzheimer's disease among others. A related study found out cancer patients who did alternate day fasting realize better cure rates, which reduced cases of deaths.

Besides all the above benefits, intermittent fasting is also easy to follow given that it makes your day much simpler. For instance, after waking up, you don't have to prepare breakfast but only require a cup of water to kick start the day.

When you're eating one less meal, you're able to plan and prepare less food, which saves time and resources. This simplicity has made intermittent fasting, an effective strategy for weight loss particularly in obese adults.

With all these benefits you stand to benefit, I am sure you are excited to get started. The good thing is that you have a variety of intermittent fasting techniques that you can choose. In the following chapters, we will look at 7 intermittent fasting techniques and how to choose one that is best suited for your needs.

5. INTERMITTENT FASTING TECHNIQUES

The reason why fasting works for many dieters is because it has different techniques and can also be modified to suit any lifestyle. All approved methods of intermittent fasting stipulate how long you'd fast and the recommended diet to adapt during the feeding phase. As a beginner in fasting, you simply need to consider your current lifestyle and personal goals before you decide the type of intermittent fasting to adapt. Though there are many techniques to follow, lets discus seven of the most popular intermittent fasting techniques and how each of them works:

1. Alternate-Day Fasting

This diet suits disciplined eaters who have a specific goal weight. Created by James Johnson, the plan recommends that dieters eat a little amount of food or no food for 1 day and then eat normally the following day.

The diet works on the belief that alternating calorie intake can activate the SIRT1 gene, which boots fat metabolism and inhibits storage of fat. If on low calorie diet, let's say that of 2,000 calories daily, then you should eat 1/5th of your daily calories the first day. This translated to around 400 calories, which is a significant calorie cut especially for beginners.

To fight hunger during low-calorie days, you can opt for meal replacement shakes that are rich in essential nutrients. Try sipping the shakes in the entire day as opposed to splitting them into smaller meals. These shakes are however restricted to the first 2 days of the diet, to help you get adapted to low-calorie diet. For those who workout, you can reduce your weight-lifting exercises if you find it harder to hit the gym on the low calorie days, or save the sweat sessions for the normal calorie days.

According to reports, alternate day fasting can help you lose about 2 1/2 pounds of weight in a week especially if you cut calories intake by **20 to 35 percent. However, critics argue that as the diet is easy to follow, it can motivate dieters to binge eat on "normal eating"** days. If that's your worry, you can control binge eating on normal calorie days by scheduling meals beforehand, in order to meet the goal weight.

2. The Warrior Diet

Love Yourself and Intermittent Fasting

Developed by Ori Hofmekler, the fasting plan is suited for people who like to follow strict rules, i.e. those dedicated or devoted. On this fasting plan, you are supposed to fast for 20 hours a day while training, and then eat one large meal at night. Actually, the creator of the diet was of the view that human beings are nocturnal eaters, specifically adapted to eat at night. While it may sound awkward, night eating is believed to help the body synthesize hormones and facilitate fat-burning during daytime. As opposed to many fasting plans, the warrior diet also recommends the type of foods to eat. Such dietary recommendations help you to feed the body with the nutrients it requires to be in sync with your circadian rhythms.

The initial fasting phase of the diet is concerned with 'under-eating' or not eating at all. However, for beginners, you can eat some raw veggies or fruits and a little protein during the 20 hours fast. This restricted eating is designed to maximize the flight response of your sympathetic nervous system, to boost energy, promote alertness and burn fat. After the 20-hours fast, you are allowed to eat; but you should begin with food groups such as veggies, the proteins and if need be eat fats much later. In case you finish the suggested food groups and you're not yet full, you are allowed to eat little amount of carbs. The 4 hours eating phase is designed to help the body to recover, and promote relaxation while absorbing the nutrients required for growth and repair.

The main advantage of warrior diet fasting plan is that you're allowed to eat a few snacks now and again so you can keep hunger at bay. And according to followers of the diet, you tend to achieve higher energy levels as well as increased fat loss. However, the strict diet plan can interfere with eating patterns especially if in places like social **gatherings. Those who don't like eating large meals late at night can find it harder to follow the guidelines on food to eat or eating in the order recommended.**

3. Eat Stop Eat Fasting Plan

Developed by Brad Pilon, the fasting plan basically targets healthy eaters who need an extra boost for weight loss. The plan revolves all about moderation i.e. you can eat all food types you want but in controlled amounts.

Here you are required to fast for up to 24 hours 1-2 times a week, in what is referred to as

"24 break from eating". During the fasting period, no eating food is allowed save for calorie-free beverages like water. Once the fasting period is concluded, you begin to eat normally without need to compensate for the time spent fasting. You can choose to break the fast with a big meal or just enjoy a healthy afternoon snack if this is what works for you. The timing is extremely flexible thus you can adjust it as per your preferences.

The Eat Stop Eat approach can help you reduce calorie intake without need to limit what you eat or count calories. Another benefit is that the plan is flexible in that you can start fasting for fewer hours than recommended 24 and then gradually increase the duration. For instance, you can begin the fast when busy; say on a day when you have no food or specific dinning obligations. Another benefit is that foods aren't restricted on the types of foods to eat or avoid, and that you don't have to count calories.

On the downside, you might find it difficult to manage 24 hours of fasting particularly when beginning the fasting. Within this period, you can experience mood changes and symptoms such as fatigue, headache, being anxious or sick especially for women. According to research, fasting can cause hormonal imbalance as starvation triggers hunger hormones and thus binge eating. It can also halt ovulation, stop menstrual cycle and reduce fertility by shrinking the ovaries. To some dieters, long period of dieting can make it more tempting to binge eat after fast and this can hamper weight loss.

However, you can improve body composition and lose weight with the plan, by including a number of workouts, especially resistance training. Another drawback is that though you can prevent binge eating (read over-eating), it requires self-control and usually takes time.

4. Lean-Gains Plan

As the name suggests, this fasting plan is designed to help gym goers who intend to loss body fat while building muscle. Created by Martain Berkhan, Lean-gains suggest that men should fast for 16 hours and women for about 14 hours daily.

In the fast period, you're not required to consume calories but there's an exception in sugar-free gum, diet soda, calorie-free sweeteners and black coffee preferably with a splash of milk. After breaking the fast, you can feed for the remaining 8-10 hours depending on your activity level.

The type of food to eat during the eating period largely depends on your workout, since you'll need higher carbs supply than fat when working out. However, protein content should be relatively higher say 1-1.5 grams of protein per body pound but this also depends on your activity level and gender.

As a starter, you may find it easier to fast from night to morning, and then continue with the fast 6 hours after bed. Although lean-gains plan can work for anyone or workout lifestyle, it's important to maintain a regular feeding window. While this may not seem important, it can help prevent your bodily hormones from getting off balance. While eating is not restricted, your calories must come from whole and unprocessed foods as these supply energy without causing sugar crashes. In some cases, you

can take a meal replacement bar or a little amount of protein shake that has no added sugars. As a beginner, you may find this plan favorable since you can eat at whichever time you choose and healthy food too within the feeding period. With a little patience, beginners can comfortably adapt to the lifestyle just like the ordinary 3 meals a day plan. However, lean-gains fasting plan has restrictions on what to eat particularly when working-out. While this helps to maximize muscle gains, some dieters find the plan strict especially when it comes to scheduling meals around workouts.

5. Fat Loss Forever

Just like the lean-gains, this fasting plan is designed to cater for gym goers who enjoy having a few cheat days. Designed by Dan Go and John Romaniello, the fasting plan allows you to enjoy a cheat day each week, although followed by a whopping 36 hours of fasting!

The diet work on the research finding that states that 36 hours of fasting boosts metabolism and accelerates weight loss. After the one-and-a half days of fasting, the remainder of 7-day cycle is divided between various fasting protocols.

For instance, you can choose Alternate Day Fasting or the Warriors Diet for that matter! This fat-loss fasting plan allows you to follow a 7-day program so that the body can achieve maximum fat loss. Particularly if on a busy program, the long fast facilitates you to focus on productivity and curb occasional cravings.

If fasting for such long is hard for you, you can download or purchase training programs designed to help maximize fat loss. While having a cheat day could be a cool idea, it can motivate you to binge eat on unhealthy snacks that can hamper weight loss goals. Worse still, the plan suggests a 36-hour long fasting schedule that can be uncomfortable for most people.

6. The 5:2 Fast Diet

This is an easy to follow fasting plan that was coined by Michael Mosley, a British doctor and journalist. As its name suggests, it involves eating regularly for 5 days and then fasting for 2 days in a week.

On fasting day, women are required to eat 500 calories in a day while men are advised to consume 600 calories. The calories can be eaten any time of the day, whether as a single meal or spread in the entire day. You're also free to choose the days to fast as far as you involve at least one non-fasting day in between. For instance, you can decide to fast on Thursday and Monday while eating 2-3 small meals of up to 600 calories. You can eat foods such as soups as these enhance satiety and are low in calories compared to actual ingredients that make them. On normal eating days, focus on whole and healthy foods especially those with high protein and fiber to facilitate weight loss. Here you can eat natural yoghurt with berries, cauliflower rice, baked or boiled eggs, grilled meat, tea, black coffee or a generous portion of veggies. To come up with your fasting plan, you'll need to experiment whatever works for you.

7. The 2-Day Fast

As compared to other fasting plans where you fast for occasional 1 day, here you do a 2 days or 48-hour fast once every few months. This means that you'll need to go to bed hungry not for one day but for two full days!

While you could be scared of hunger, the body normally enters into nutritional ketosis where it burns stored fat for energy. To your surprise, once accustomed to the fast, you hardly become hungry as ketosis keeps you going. And if afraid of burning muscle, rest assured that increased fat metabolism and levels of HGH hormone will hinder muscle loss. For beginners, you may need to begin with a 24 hours fast before attempting the 2-day fast. Then ensure that you eat dinner the previous night say between 6-8 pm. After waking up the next morning, simply drink water to stay hydrated throughout the day. At 10 o'clock, drink a cup of green tea and later a cup of black coffee around noon, or instead take some mineral water. Ensure that you're busy the entire day and avoid encounter with foods that trigger cravings such as sweet snacks. Continue taking water until evening and then some decaf coffee or herbal tea for dinner. By now, you should be ready to fall asleep without feeling any hunger; and ready to progress with day two of fasting! With practice, you'll find it easier to manage even longer than 48 hours of fasting without any negative side effects. However, health experts warn that intermittent fasting is not for everyone. For this reason, you should consult a doctor before changing your diet patterns especially if you suffer from any health conditions. You also need to consider your current lifestyle and personal goals before you decide the type of intermittent fasting to adapt. To guide you on possible fasting plan to consider, these following tips can help a lot:

How to Choose Best Fasting Technique

If healthy, managing a fast is an easy thing as far as you can retrain your body to burn fat for fuel and lose weight. Since it harder to burn fat in cases where the body accesses other sources of fuel, you should choose a technique that focuses on fewer meals that are timed to occur closely together.

You also need to eat only the real foods when it comes to eating phase, say organic produce and pastured eggs, meat and dairy.

Any fasting technique can apply here as except Fat Loss Forever plan as it suggests that you include a few cheat days. Simply cut out any sugary or processed foods such as sweets, chocolate, crisps and fizzy drinks.

But when it comes to food choices, it's advisable to consume food groups based on the type of fasting you adopt. Start by slowly withdrawing from specific foods or simply replace them with healthier or low-calorie options. For instance, you can swap the shortening or butter with coconut oil and schedule those Pop-tarts for post-workout. Also stock healthy oatcakes, unsalted rice cakes, fruit juice, unsweetened popcorn and healthy fruits. After 2-3 weeks, you can then choose to eat at specific times, say from 10 a.m-8 p.m. Once accustomed with the eating plan, you can fully embark on 16-18 hours fasting plan or alternate day fasting.

Love Yourself and Intermittent Fasting

The intermittent fasting technique that you choose should depend on your activity level, work program and the availability of food. For instance, body builders should choose Lean-Gains or Fast Loss Forever plans while non-gym goers can choose Eat Stop Diet or the 5:2 fasting plan. If busy throughout the day or unable to access food, you can try out the Warrior diet that promotes 4-hours night eating window. If ready to try something more challenging, then a 48-72 hour fasting can help you gain more in terms of weight loss. If seeking to lose weight, choose a fasting technique that can accommodate exercise. Alternatively, adopt a fitness program that is based on cardio, yoga or interval training. Being in a training program facilitates alternate periods of intense activity with bursts of slower recovery. To begin with, try 20-30 minutes of bike riding, walking or swimming to rev your metabolism and thus burn more calories. With interval training, you can develop leaner muscles to further rev the metabolism; to assist you break that weight loss plateau.

Regardless of the fasting technique that you choose, it's recommendable to not eat food but rather drink plenty of water, tea and coffee to remain hydrated. Water can serve as a good substitute for occasional snacks as it contains no calories or added sugars. To help sweeten and make water tasty, consider adding a little amount of stevia or lemon juice. Water also helps you remain hydrated and supercharges various metabolic activities among them digestion and removal of toxins from your body. In case you find it easier to fast for 2-3 weeks, consider fasting more often preferably fasting longer on weekends.

So how can you easily succeed with intermittent fasting? These 4 guidelines can be much helpful:

6. TIPS TO SUCCEED WITH FASTING & CONCLUSION

1. Don't start too ambitious

It's a hard thing to transit from binge eating or following a regular diet of junk food into a few meals in a day or no meal at all for 1-2 days. Even for dieters who now eat one meal in a day, remember they never started like that. You need to first skip your breakfast or dinner, do without lunch for at least 16 hours or 20 hours of fast.

Do not be too harsh on yourself, and don't' be overly ambitious. While it may appear easy to first, a few of dieters take days or weeks to manage a 24-48 hours of total fasting.

Also know that setting short-term achievable goals can play a big role in fighting stress that may interrupt your progress. A short term goal may include something like a lean and healthy breakfast every day within one week.

2. Don't be afraid of hunger

Understand that hunger is totally a normal part of life and that a few hours of fast can't eat away your muscles. Even with 16-48 hours of fast, you can still manage ordinary workout routines and build bigger muscles.

Furthermore, you don't have to worry on which time you eat food as far as it's within the feeding window. Some dieters eat a single meal in a day at around 3-4 pm, a meal that serves as dinner and then survive on water and tea.

In case you feel hungry before or after dinner, try eating few raw veggies or some bit of ice cream.

3. Cope with cravings

In those instances when food cravings strike, just appreciate them without allowing yourself to get distracted or rather fulfill them. Try getting yourself busy through trying out a more involving task, visit your friend or go for a walk.

Cravings do go away within 15-60 minutes of getting into more productive ventures. If not successful, take a few satiating drinks such as soups, water or tea and then consider eating more veggies during the feeding window. Veggies are delicious and tasty when served with brown rice or other whole food. Choose high fiber veggies topped with whole grains to fight hunger.

Such dietary combination also helps to slow down the absorption of glucose into your blood.

4. Get enough nutrients

You can also take multivitamins or 5-8 grams of amino acids such as branched chain amino acids (BCAAs). These support weight loss by strengthening your body cells and muscles, bones and supplying required energy. For instance, vitamin B helps your body cells make protein, release energy and to manufacture serotonin, a brain chemical. Get vitamin B from fat-free dairy products, soy products, salmon, sardines, lean meat, eggs and fat-free peanut butter.

With these tips and strong will at heart, you can surely overcome any barrier as far as fasting is concerned. But in case you develop negative hormonal imbalance symptoms such as fatigue, headaches, bloating, depression or irregular periods, stop fasting. It's wise to do so as such symptoms may accelerate it to an eating disorder or other serious condition.

Conclusion

Tip: To effectively burn fat and build muscle, carb cycling can really be helpful so you can find a blend of intermittent fasting and carb cycling. When carb intake is low, the body is forced to use body fat as source of energy. However, the body still require specific amount of carbs to facilitate nervous and brain functions. Thus for gym goers, try to up the carb intake to at least 50 grams to replenish your glycogen stores. Ensure that you consume enough amounts of proteins and fats while not limiting intake of carbohydrates below 50 grams. With the correct approach, you should reap benefits of intermittent fasting within no time!

Hey! Do you mind giving your feedback on Amazon by rating and reviewing my book.

I would really appreciate that.

My Other Books available across the platforms in e-book, paperback and audible versions:

1. Love Yourself: 21 day plan for learning "Self-Love" to cultivate self-worth ,self-belief, self-confidence & happiness

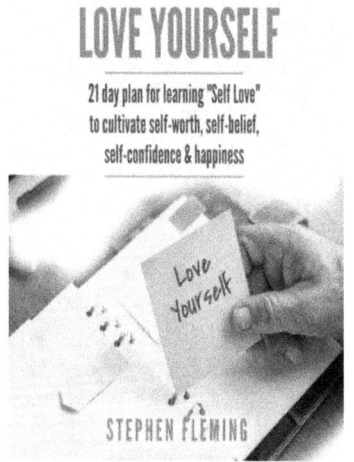

2. Intermittent Fasting: 7 effective techniques of Intermittent Fasting

3. Love Yourself and Intermittent Fasting

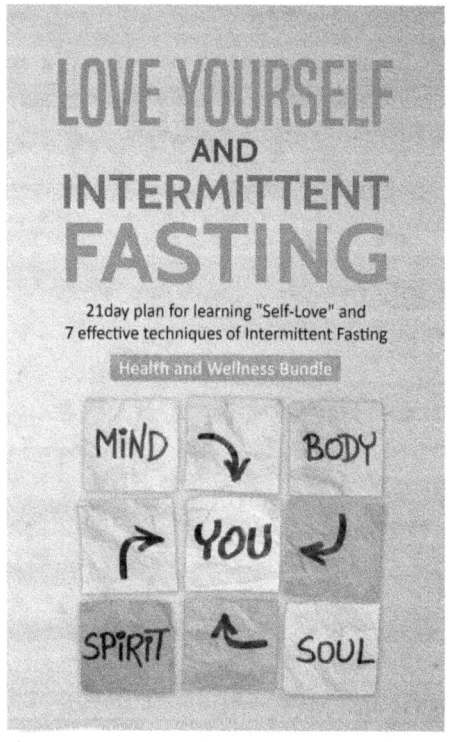

4. Blockchain Technology : Introduction to Blockchain Technology and its impact on Business Ecosystem

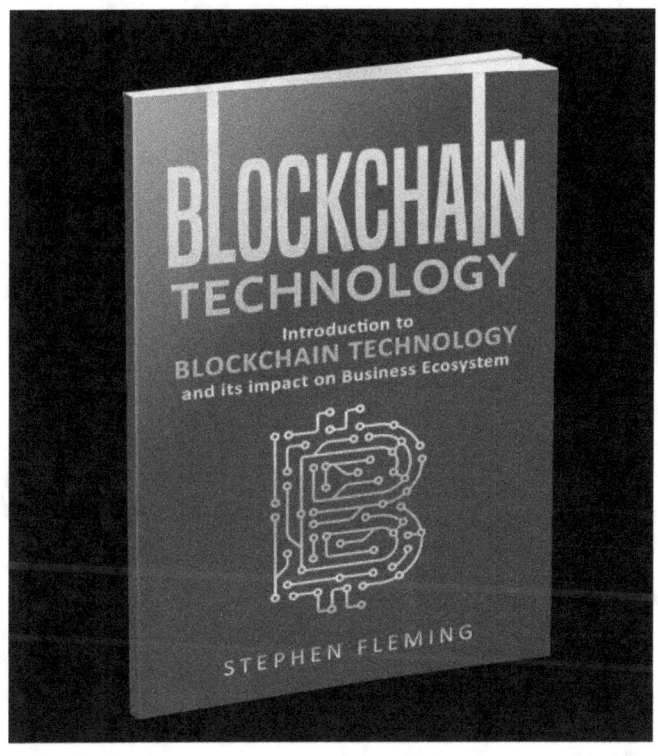

5. DevOps Handbook: Introduction to DevOps and its impact on Business Ecosystem

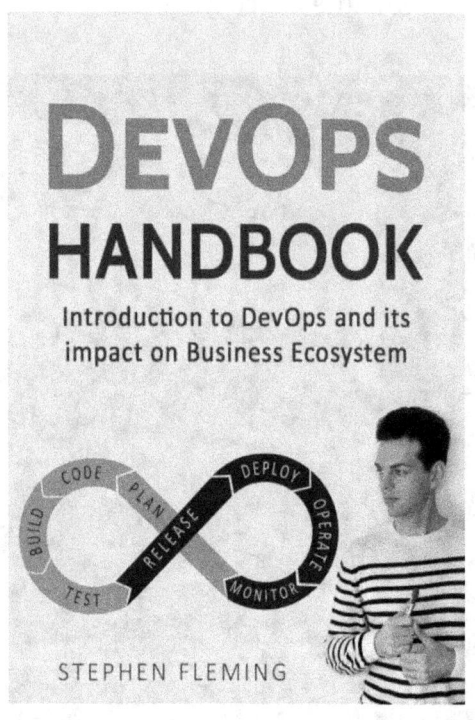

6. Blockchain Technology & DevOps: Introduction and impact on Business Ecosystem

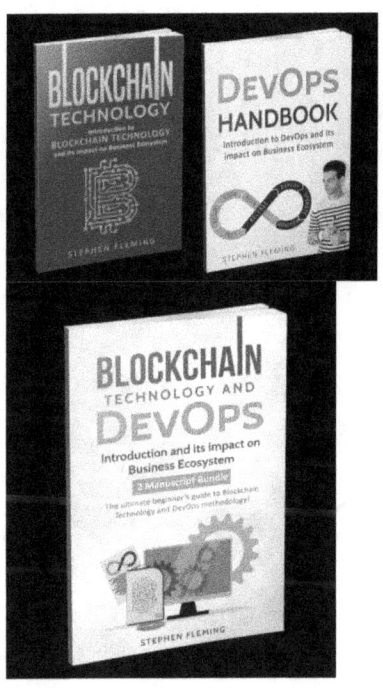

** If you prefer audible versions of these books, I have few free coupons, drop me a mail at: **valueadd2life@gmail.com.** If available, I would mail you the same.

www.ingramcontent.com/pod-product-compliance
Lightning Source LLC
LaVergne TN
LVHW011853060526
838200LV00054B/4312